CROCK POT COOKBOOK 2021

2021

SUPER TASTY RECIPES

JIMMY FORTE

Table of Contents

Vegetable Eggs Supreme

INGREDIENTS

- 8 eggs

- 3/4 cup milk

- 8 ounces shredded Cheddar cheese

- 2 cups chopped cooked broccoli

- 1 cup sliced mushrooms

- salt and pepper to taste

PREPARATION

1. Beat eggs; add milk and beat together. Pour mixture into greased crockpot or slow cooker. Add cheese, broccoli, mushrooms, salt & pepper. Cook on HIGH 1 1/2 to 2 1/2 hours.

Wild Rice Casserole

INGREDIENTS

- 1 1/2 cups uncooked long-grained rice

- 1/2 cup uncooked wild rice

- 1 envelope dry onion soup mix

- 1 teaspoon dried parsley flakes, or 1 tablespoon chopped fresh parsley

- 4 cups water

- 1 bunch green onions, chopped, about 8 green onions

- 8 oz. sliced fresh or canned mushrooms

- 1/4 cup butter, melted

PREPARATION

1. Combine all ingredients. Pour into lightly greased slow cooker. Cover and cook on HIGH for 2 1/2 hours, stirring occasionally.

Southwest Chicken Soup

Ingredients:

- 1 litre of chicken broth (more if you want it thinner instead of thick)

- 1-2 boneless chicken breasts, raw

- 1 can black beans, drained and rinsed (or you can make your own)

- 1 can sweet corn (or equivalent frozen), drained

- 1 can diced (no salt added) tomatoes

- 1 bunch fresh cilantro, about a cup roughly chopped

- 4 green onions, chopped

- 1 pepper of your choice (jalapeno, habanero, scotch bonnet), seeds removed and chopped

- Spices:

- Garlic Powder

- Cumin

-
Chili Powder

-
Smoked Paprika (optional)

-
Salt and Pepper

Method:

1.
Turn your crock pot on high if you want it done in 3-4 hours, low if you want to let it cook all day.

2.
Add all ingredients above except the chicken breasts. Add your spices. I would suggest starting with a teaspoon of the spices and adjust the amount of each according to your taste preference.

3.
Stir all ingredients together and place your chicken breast(s) on top. Cook until your chicken is cooked through and tender.

4.
Once your chicken has been cooked through, remove the chicken and shred it.

5.
Then place the chicken back in the crock pot. Do your final tasting and spicing and enjoy.

Mark's Homemade Chili

Ingredients:

-

1 lb ground beef, cooked, drained

-

1 large onion

-

3 cans dark red kidney beans, drained

-

2 cans dice tomatoes (we get whatever seasoned ones they have at Kroger at the time)

-

1 large can of tomato sauce

-

Worcestershire sauce – 5 shakes or more. We shake whatever feels good at the time. We like lots of this.

-

Salt and pepper to taste

-

3 t chili powder

To Make:

1.

Throw it all in the Crock pot and cook on low for 6-8 hours. We might season more as we go depending on if we are around or not to do so.

Chicken Tortilla Soup

What you need:

- 1 pound boneless chicken breasts

- 1 can diced tomatoes

- ½ C chunky salsa

- 1 C homemade enchilada sauce

- 1 medium onion, chopped

- 1 can black beans, drained (optional)

- 2 cloves garlic, chopped

- 4 C chicken broth

- 2 t cumin

- 1 t chili powder

- 1 T lemon juice

- 1 bay leaf

What to do:

1.

Set crockpot to high heat

2.

Add raw chopped chicken into crockpot as well as the chopped onion and broth, stir (you can add whole breasts and shred once fully cooked)

3.

Add remaining ingredients and set crockpot to low heat

4.

Let cook for about 3-4 hours depending on your crockpot

5.

Top soup with sour cream, cilantro and avocado slices

6.

Serve with tortilla chips and Enjoy!

Cincinnati Chili

Ingredients

⬚

2 pounds ground meat

⬚

1 large onion, minced

⬚

1 teaspoon garlic powder

⬚

1 cup (8 ounces) tomato sauce

⬚

2 cups water

⬚

1 teaspoon Worcestershire sauce

⬚

1 tablespoon vinegar

⬚

1 teaspoon salt

⬚

½ teaspoon black pepper

⬚

4+ teaspoons chili powder (we used 4 tablespoons, but some claim that's too much)

⬚

1 teaspoon cinnamon

?

½ teaspoon allspice

?

1 ½ cups cooked kidney beans

?

Cheese

?

Noodles

Method

1.
In a skillet, brown the ground meat.

2.
Pour into 5 quart crock.

3.
Stir in onion, garlic powder, tomato sauce, water, Worcestershire, vinegar, salt, pepper, chili powder, cinnamon, and allspice.

4.
Cover and cook on low for 8 hours.

5.
1 hour before done, add kidney beans.

6.
Boil desired pasta.

7.
Layer noodles in bowl, add chili, and top with cheese.

Curried Sweet Potato and Carrot Soup

Ingredients

- 2 large sweet potatoes, peeled and cut into chunks

- 2 cups baby carrots (almost 1 pound)

- 1 small onion, chopped

- ¾ teaspoon curry powder

- ½ teaspoon salt

- ½ teaspoon black pepper

- ½ teaspoon ground cinnamon

- ¼ teaspoon ground ginger

- 4 cups chicken broth

- 1 tablespoon maple syrup

- ¾ cup cream

Instructions

1.

Place potatoes, carrots, onion, curry powder, salt, pepper, cinnamon and ginger in a greased crock pot.

2.

Add chicken broth and stir.

3.

Cover and cook on low for 7-8 hours.

4.

Puree soup in a blender a few cups at a time or use an immersion blender. Stir in maple syrup and cream.

5.

Serve.

Turkey Sausage and Red Bean Stew

Ingredients

- 1 pound turkey sausage (browned)
- 2 cups cooked red beans or 1 can (15 ounces) small red beans
- 1/2 cup brown rice (uncooked)
- 1 cup water
- 1 1/2 cups corn (frozen or canned)
- 2 cups tomato juice
- 1/2 cup chopped sweet green pepper (more if you like)
- salt and pepper, to taste

Instructions

1.

Combine all ingredients in a slow cooker. Cook on low setting for 6 hours. This stew is great served with hot cornbread and a glass of milk. It is also gluten free – a bonus for those of you with GF needs! Makes 6-8 servings.

Chicken Noodle Soup

Ingredients

- 5 cups chicken broth (or bouillon)
- 5-6 cups water
- 2 cups carrots, sliced thin
- 1 cup celery, sliced thin
- 1 small onion, finely chopped
- 2 garlic cloves, minced
- 2 tsp parsley flakes
- 1/2 tsp dried basil
- 1 tsp pepper
- 2-3 lbs boneless skinless chicken breast
- 1 cup dry egg noodles

Directions

1.

Mix all ingredients except the noodles into the crockpot pot. Keep chicken breast whole (or use pre-cooked, cut up or shredded chicken) and cut up or shred before adding in noodles during the last 30 minutes of cooking. Cook on high 4 hours, then turn to low until ready to serve.

Lentil Vegetable Soup

Ingredients

☐

2 cups dried lentils, rinsed and looked over

☐

2 cans diced tomatoes (14.5 ounces each)

☐

1 cup chopped onion

☐

2 stalks celery, chopped

☐

1 cup chopped carrot

☐

1 can chilies (4 ounce size)

☐

5 cups chicken broth (or replace with vegetable stock)

☐

1 teaspoon salt

☐

1 teaspoon oregano

☐

1 teaspoon thyme

☐

½ teaspoon garlic powder

☐

¼ teaspoon pepper

Directions

1.

Combine all ingredients in a 4-5 quart crock pot.

2.

Cover and cook on low for 8-9 hours or until lentils are tender.

Mexican Chicken Chili

▢

1 shredded rotisserie chicken or 3 cups shredded chicken breasts

▢

2 cups black beans

▢

2 cups pinto beans

▢

1 cup frozen corn

▢

3-4 chopped zucchini (I LOVE zucchini so I put a ton in)

▢

5 cups chicken broth

▢

2 cups chunky salsa (mild or hot depending on taste)

▢

1 8oz can tomato sauce

Directions

1.
Combine in the crock pot and cook for 7-8 hours on low.

Mexican Soup

Meat:

- 1 lb ground beef, sausage, or pork (browned)

- or 2 cups shredded chicken, cooked

Must-have veggies:

- 1 onion sliced (half moon and big dice)

- 3 garlic cloves, minced (or smashed if you want to pull them out later)

-

Optional Veggies

- 1 large zucchini, large dice or (2 cups shredded if you preserved)

- 3 celery stalks, chopped

- 1 bunch of asparagus (chopped)

The rest:

- 2 sweet potatoes, peeled and diced

- 1 can diced tomatoes (in juice)

- 1 quart chicken stock

- 1 6 oz can tomato paste + 4 cups of water

- 2 T Maple Syrup

- Cumin (about 1T)

- Chili Powder (about 1/2T)

- 1/2 T basil

- 1/2 T oregano

- 1 T salt

- 1/2 T pepper

Method:

1.
Layer all of the ingredients up to (and including) the chicken stock.

2.
Combine remaining ingredients in mixing bowl.

3.
Mix well and pour over crock pot ingredients.

4.
Stir gently and seal 'er up!

5.
Cook on low for 4-6 hours.

Moroccan Chicken Stew

Modified from Victoria Taylor's Gourmet Blog

- ½ pound baby carrots

- 1 cup chopped green peppers

- 1 cup chopped onion

- 2 tablespoons lemon juice

- 1 teaspoon ginger

- 1 medium butternut squash, cut into 2 inch cubes

- 1 can (15 ounces) chickpeas, drained

- 2 14.5 ounce cans diced tomatoes

- 1 ½ pounds boneless, skinless chicken thighs or chicken breast

- 3 tablespoons Moroccan seasoning (homemade version here)

Method:

1.

In a 5-6 quart crock pot, combine carrots, peppers, onion, lemon juice, ginger, squash, chickpeas, and tomatoes.

2.

Sprinkle with 2 tablespoons Moroccan seasoning. Toss veggies to coat.

3.

Lay chicken thighs on top of veggies. Sprinkle with remaining seasoning.

4.

Cover and cook on low for 8 hours. Salt and pepper to taste.

5.

Remove chicken and shred. Stir back into stew. Or serve thighs whole on top of veggies in a soup bowl.

Vegetable Beef Soup

- 1 pound ground beef (venison or turkey would also work)

- 1 ½ cups cooked beans of your choice (I like kidney) or 1 can beans, rinsed and drained

- 28 ounces diced tomatoes, undrained

- 12 ounces frozen mixed vegetables

- 3 cups beef broth

- 1 teaspoon salt

- 1 teaspoon dried onion

- 1 teaspoon oregano

- ½ teaspoon thyme

- ½ teaspoon pepper

Method:

1.

Brown ground meat in skillet. Drain.

2.

Add to 4 quart crock pot with remaining ingredients.

3.

Cover and cook on low for 8 hours.

Yield: 4-6 servings

WINTER SQUASH AND SAUSAGE SOUP

Check your sausage for "illegal" ingredients like sugar and gluten. I like Applegate Farm brand.

You can also make this recipe on a stove top if you're in a hurry. But I like the long, lazy style of a slow cooker.

Source: Erin at Plan to Eat

Course: Allergen-Free Soup and Stew

Serves: 6

Ingredients

-
2 Tbs butter

-
1 leek thinly sliced

-
2 cloves garlic minced

-
1 small butternut squash peeled and diced

-
1 1/2 c mushrooms chopped

-
1 Tbs fresh sage chopped

-
1 tsp fresh rosemary chopped

-

1 pound Italian sausage sliced and cut into quarters

-

salt to taste

-

1/4 tsp white pepper

-

4 cups chicken broth homemade if possible

-

2 cups leafy greens kale, chard, collards, etc.

Directions

1.

Turn a slow cooker on high, and melt the butter in the crock while it warms up. Add the leeks and garlic; replace the lid and allow to soften–about 20-30 minutes. Add the remaining veggies, herbs, and the sausage. Replace the lid and allow to soften–about 30-45 minutes. Season with salt and pepper. Add the chicken broth and allow to cook on high for 6-8 hours.

2.

30 minutes before serving, switch the heat to the low setting and add the greens. Replace the lid and allow the soup to simmer until the greens have melted into the soup.

French Lentil & Brown Rice Soup

Ingredients

- 6 cups of organic vegetable broth (make your own and save money)

- 2 cups filtered water

- 1 ½ cup of organic French lentils, rinsed

- 2 medium organic carrots, peeled and diced

- 1 organic onion, finely chopped

- 2 stalks of organic celery, diced

- 5 tablespoons of uncooked organic brown rice

- 1 strip of Kombu seaweed (adds essential minerals, vitamins, and trace elements to your soup)

- 2 cloves of organic garlic, minced

- 1 teaspoon of herbs de Provence or 1 teaspoon of thyme

- ½ teaspoon of sea salt

Method:

1.

Stir together broth, lentils, carrots, onion, celery, rice, kombu, garlic, herbs, and salt in the crock pot slow cooker. Cover and cook on Low for 8 hours or High for 5 hours. Spoon out the kombu and serve.

Tomato Soup

INGREDIENTS

- 2 lbs tomatoes (chopped and peeled) or a 28 oz jar diced tomatoes (unseasoned, with juice)

- 2 cups chopped yellow onion

- 1/4 tsp salt

- 1/8 tsp pepper

o tbsp minced garlic- 2 cloves

- 1/8 tsp red pepper flakes (for a spicy little kick)

- 1/4 tsp smoked paprika

- 1/2 tsp dried basil

- 1 tbsp honey (I like raw)

- 1 cup chicken broth (homemade or a good quality low sodium store-bought)

o bay leaves

-

for garnish: fresh basil leaves and Greek yogurt, optional

Method:

1.

Roughly chop onion and toss in a large pan with some olive oil over medium heat Sprinkle with salt and pepper, stir, and let cook for a few minutes. Meanwhile, mince the garlic.

2.

Let cook for a couple of minutes, until softened and fragrant

3.

Then add the tomatoes (with their juices) to the pan

4.

Add smoked paprika and red pepper flakes- 1/8 tsp of red pepper flakes

5.

Add remaining herbs and spices... And honey

6.

Add to Crock Pot

7.

Add chicken broth and bay leaves

8.

Set on low for about 4 hours

9.

When it's done, stir and taste for flavors- depending on your personal preferences you may want to add salt etc.

10.

Remove bay leaves

11.

Either use an immersion blender or pour soup into a blender and blend until smooth

12.

The level of chunkiness is up to you- some people like their soups totally smooth,

13.

others like some texture... I left some tomato chunks in there because I like the texture

14.

Voila... we have soup!

15.

Top with Greek yogurt, fresh basil, and if you have them, little cherry tomatoes...

16.

Serve with grilled cheese, crackers, or eat just as is!

17.

Enjoy!!

Texas Calico Chili

Ingredients

- 1 ½ pounds stew beef

- ½ cup onion, chopped

- 2 cans (14.5 ounce) diced tomatoes

- 6 ounce can tomato paste mixed with water to make 1 cup

- 1 can (4.5 ounce) chopped green chilies

- 1 ½ cups cooked black beans

- 1 ½ cups cooked white beans (navy or great northern)

- ½ teaspoon onion powder

- ½ teaspoon garlic powder

- 2 teaspoons chili powder

- 2 teaspoons cumin

Method:

1.

Combine all ingredients in 4-5 quart crock pot. Stir well.

2.

Cover and cook on low for 8-10 hours. Serve with cornbread.

Homemade Chili

Ingredients

- pound ground meat (we prefer venison)

- onion

- green pepper

- 1/2 tbsp ground mustard seed

- tbsp chili powder

- 1 tbsp hot sauce

- 1 can red kidney beans (or two cups dry/cooked red kidney beans)

- 1 can black beans (or two cups dry/cooked black beans)

- 1 can (8 oz) tomato sauce

- 1 can (28 oz) diced tomatoes

- Salt & pepper to taste (I do 1 tsp of each)

Method:

1.

Brown meat, drain, return to pan, and mix in diced green peppers and onions. Once finished, add to crockpot with all spices, beans (preferably undrained), tomato sauce, diced tomatoes, salt, and pepper. Cook in crockpot on low for 6-8 hours. Serve alongside cornbread or potatoes. Yum!

Chili

Ingredients

- 2 cups dry beans OR 4 cups cooked/canned beans

- 1 pound ground venison, antelope, or beef

- 2 tablespoons coconut oil or bacon fat

- 1 medium onion, chopped finely

- 6 cloves of garlic, minced

- 2 1/2 cups crushed or diced tomatoes with juice (approx. 2 cans)

- 3 cups broth or stock

- 1/4 cup chili powder

- 2 T. dried oregano

- 2 T. cumin

- 2 t. sea salt

- 1/2 t. black pepper

-

Garnish: sour cream and shredded cheese (optional)

Instructions

1.

Soak beans overnight

2.

Next morning: brown your meat

3.

Add browned meat to crockpot, add coconut oil or bacon fat

4.

Saute the onions until tender, then add the garlic and cook until soft

5.

Add to slow cooker

6.

Drain and rinse soaked beans and add them to the mixture

7.

Add tomatoes, broth, and all of the seasonings except the salt (Adding salt too soon prevents beans from getting soft)

8.

I set slow cooker on high and let it go 6-7 hours, but crockpots vary, so plan according to how your appliance works

9.

Add salt when beans are done cooking

10.

We like to garnish with sour cream and shredded cheddar cheese

Gluten-Free Taco Soup

Ingredients

- 1lb boneless skinless chicken breast, cooked and shredded

- 16oz homemade salsa

- 14oz whole kernel corn, drained

- 2 cups soaked and cooked black beans (or 14 oz. can, rinsed and drained)

- 2 cups soaked and cooked kidney beans (or 14 oz. can, rinsed and drained)

- 6oz tomato paste

- quart chicken stock

- 28oz diced tomatoes

- 1/2 cup onions, diced

- 1/2 cup red or green peppers, diced

- cloves of garlic, minced

- teaspoon chili powder

- tablespoons taco seasoning (or 1 store-bought pkg.)

- 8oz sour cream (optional)

Directions

1.

I love this part! Throw everything but the sour cream in a crockpot. (I use a 6 qt. crockpot and this recipe nearly fills it.) Turn it on low for about 3 hours.

2.

Add the homemade sour cream and stir it well. Keep soup on low for about another 30 min. or until it is fully heated.

3.

Serve with extra homemade sour cream and tortilla chips if desired.

Tuscan Kale and White Bean Soup

Ingredients:

In the Crock

- 2 quarts water

- 2 cups, dried, great northern white beans, soaked for two nights

- 2 medium carrots, roughly chopped

- 2 ribs celery, roughly chopped

- 1/2 large yellow onion, roughly chopped

- 3 medium potatoes, peeled and chopped into bite sized pieces

- 3 tbls extra virgin olive oil

- 2 tsp onion salt by Real Salt (sub plain salt)

On the Stovetop

- 2 tbls extra virgin olive oil

- 2 large handfuls of kale

-

4 cloves garlic

-

bean puree (in recipe below)

-

1 tsp onion salt by Real Salt (sub plain salt)

Method:

In the Crock

1.
Soak your beans, preferably for two nights, rinsing and changing the water after each day. This will ensure that your beans become soft and tender.

2.
Drain and rinse your beans.

3.
In a large crockpot add the water, beans, carrots, celery, onion, potatoes, 3 tbls extra virgin olive oil, and salt. Mix together well and cook on low for 8 hours.

On the Stovetop

1.
Once the beans and vegetables are soft and tender, remove one cup of beans and one cup of broth. Make sure to replace the lid on the crockpot.

2.
Puree the beans and broth in a blender or food processor.

3.

Once the beans and the broth have been pureed, heat 2 tbls extra virgin olive oil in heavy bottomed sauce pan or cast iron skillet. Add the kale and garlic. Saute for 2-3 minutes or until the kale begins to wilt and the garlic lets out its aroma. Add the bean puree and saute for an additional 2-3 minutes or until the flavors begin to incorporate.

4.

Add the bean kale mixture back to the crock and mix through. This will add more flavor and depth to the soup. Allow to continue to cook in the crock, covered, for an additional 10 minutes.

Fried Crusty Bread

1.

To heighten the flavors of the soup, spread extra virgin olive oil on both sides of crusty bread.

2.

In a shallow frying pan or cast iron skillet heat an additional 1 tbls of extra virgin olive oil and add one clove of freshly minced or pressed garlic.

3.

Place the bread on top of the oil and garlic and allow to toast on both sides.

4.

To serve, place the bread on the bottom of a bowl, topped with the soup, and sprinkled with freshly grated parmesan or pecorino romano cheese.

Chicken Posole Stew

serves 4 – 6

Ingredients

For the stew:

-

2 bone-in chicken breasts, skin removed

-

2 (15 oz.) cans white hominy, rinsed and drained

-

3 cups good quality chicken stock

-

2 (14.5 oz.) cans of diced tomatoes

-

3 carrots, peeled and sliced into thin rounds

-

3 scallions, both green and white parts, sliced thinly

-

3 cloves of garlic, minced

-

tablespoon cumin

-

teaspoons light ancho chili powder

-

½ teaspoons Mexican oregano

-

1/8 teaspoon cayenne pepper

-

teaspoon salt, or to taste

-

½ teaspoon fresh ground black pepper

-

Optional toppings:

-

Chopped cilantro

-

Queso Fresco or other good quality Mexican cheese (Monterrey jack would work)

-

Shredded radishes (Use the large holes on your box grater)

-

Avocado

-

Sour cream

-

Tortilla chips

Method:

1.
Place chicken breasts in the bottom of the CrockPot.

2.

Put remaining ingredients in and stir the top to mix in spices.

3.

Cover and cook on low for 5 – 6 hours, or until chicken and carrots are cooked through and tender.

4.

Remove chicken from

5.

CrockPot and shred with two forks.

6.

Return chicken to CrockPot, stir to combine.

7.

Serve with toppings if desired.

Easy BBQ Sauce

Ingredients

- c. ketchup

- 1/3 c. vinegar

- 1/3 c. Worcestershire sauce

- 1/2 c. brown sugar

- tsp. salt

- tsp. mustard

Method:

1.

I placed the chicken (any bone-in kind will do; I used split breasts) in the crockpot and poured the BBQ sauce over it:

2.

I set the crockpot to cook on low for 8 hours, but it didn't take anywhere near that long. I set it going around 8:00 in the morning, and it was perfectly cooked by 12:30. If I want it to take longer, I leave the chicken (or whatever meat I'm using) frozen.

3.

BBQ in the crock pot is QUICK, aside from the time to cook in the crock pot. Five minutes max to mix the sauce and set it going, and then you can do whatever you want while the crock pot does its job!

Sloppy Joes

Ingredients

- 2 lbs ground beef

- 1 small onion, chopped

- 1 green pepper, chopped

- 1 ½ cups ketchup

- ¼ cup sucanat (or brown sugar)

- ¼ cup apple cider vinegar (white vinegar would work too)

- ¼ cup mustard

- 1 tsp Worchestershire sauce

- ½ tsp pepper

- 1 tsp salt

Method:

1.

Brown ground beef in a large skillet with the onion and green pepper.

2.

Add browned ground beef mixture along with the remaining ingredients to the crock pot. Mix well to combine.

3.

Cook on low for at least 3 hours, but up to 6 hours.

Crock Pot Style Gyros

Ingredients

☐
1 pound ground beef

☐
1 pound ground pork or turkey

☐
1 onion sliced

☐
3 cloves of garlic minced

☐
2 teaspoons Greek seasoning

Method:

1.
Place onion and garlic in the crock pot. Mix together meat and Greek seasoning. Form into two small loaves and place on top of onions and garlic, like this.

2.
Cook on low for 4-5 hours or until done

Sauce:

Ingredients

⬜

1 cucumber, peeled, seeded, and chopped

⬜

8 ounces of plain yogurt

⬜

½ teaspoon of Greek seasoning

⬜

½ teaspoon of lemon juice

⬜

½ teaspoon salt

Method:

1.

Mix together and refrigerate until you are ready to serve.

2.

Slice the meat and serve on pita or tortillas with shredded lettuce and yogurt sauce.

Barbecue Beef Brisket

Ingredients:

- 2 -3 lbs Beef Brisket

- 1 tsp Chili Powder

- ½ tsp Garlic Powder

- ½ tsp Crushed Red Pepper

- ¼ tsp Celery Seed

- 1/8 tsp Pepper

- ½ cup Ketchup

- ¼ cup Sucanat or Brown Sugar

- 2 Tbsp Apple Cider Vinegar

- 2 Tbsp Worcestershire Sauce

- ½ tsp Dry Mustard

Directions:

1.

In a small bowl mix chili powder, garlic, crushed red pepper, celery seed and pepper and rub onto meat.

2.

Place meat in crock-pot.

3.

Mix ketchup, sucanat/sugar, vinegar, Worcestershire sauce and dry mustard and pour over meat.

4.

Cover and cook on low for 8-10 hours or high for 4-5 hours.

5.

Cut thin slices along the grain or just shred it.

Beef Enchiladas

Ingredients:

-

1 ½ lb ground beef

-

1 large onion, chopped

-

4 cloves garlic, minced

-

32 ounces homemade or all-natural enchilada sauce or salsa (we like tomatillo salsa!)

-

1 cup crème fraiche (or real sour cream: ingredients should say "cream, culture")

-

1 ½ cups refried beans (homemade, if possible!)

-

2-3 cups shredded cheddar (buy good quality and shred it yourself)

-

One dozen homemade tortillas or all-natural from the store

Instructions:

1.

Brown the meat, drain and set aside.

2.

Saute the onions and garlic in butter until soft, then return the meat to the pan. Add the sauce or salsa and the crème fraiche. Simmer for 10 minutes.

3.

In a buttered crockpot, put a thin layer of sauce, then layer in this order: tortillas, refried beans, meat sauce and cheese. Repeat until all ingredients are used, ending with cheese.

4.

Cook on low 5 hours.

5.

Serve with fresh cilantro, more crème fraiche and lacto-fermented salsa.

Mexican Stew Meat

Ingredients

- 4+ onions

- 4-6 tomatillos

- 4+ peppers (any variety)

- Several Cloves of Garlic Crushed

- Salt

- Pepper

- Pounds Beef Stew Meat (or other meat of choice)

Directions:

1.

Blend all vegetables in a blender until pureed to your liking, (smooth, chunky or in between).

2.

Place the meat in the slow cooker, sprinkle with salt and pepper then pour the vegetable puree over all.

3.

Cover and cook on low for 6-8 hours.

4.

Serve in warm tortillas!

Beef and Bacon Hash

Yield: 4 servings

Prep Time: 30 min

Cook Time: 6 hours

Ingredients

- 6 cups beef broth

- 2 teaspoons onion powder

- 1 teaspoon celery salt

- 3 Tablespoons minced onions

- 1 teaspoon salt

- ½ teaspoon black pepper

- 1 (2-pound) rump roast

- 4 Idaho potatoes, peeled and halved

- 2 large carrots, peeled and halved

-

1 large onion, peeled and medium diced

-

4 slices bacon

-

8 eggs, for serving (optional)

Directions:

1.

Add the beef broth to the crock pot (See Kelly's Notes), and then stir in the onion powder, celery salt, minced onions, salt and pepper.

2.

Add the roast, potatoes and carrots to the crock pot and set it to LOW. Allow the roast and vegetables to cook in the crock pot for 6 hours, or until tender.

3.

Remove the cooked roast and vegetables from the crock pot and dice everything into bite-sized pieces. Combine the mixture with the diced white onion.

4.

Saute the bacon in a large skillet, reserving the drippings. Set the cooked bacon aside.

5.

Add the hash mixture to the skillet containing the bacon grease and and fry the hash until crispy, about 10 minutes. Chop up the bacon and add it to the skillet, tossing to combine.

6.

If desired, fry 2 eggs per person in a separate pan and serve the hash topped with the fried eggs.

Spaghetti Sauce

Ingredients

☐

2 lb bulk Italian pork sausage or ground beef

☐

2 large onions, chopped (2 cups)

☐

2 cups sliced fresh mushrooms (6 oz)

☐

3 cloves garlic, finely chopped

☐

1 can (28 oz) Muir Glen® organic diced tomatoes, undrained

☐

2 cans (15 oz each) tomato sauce

☐

1 can (6 oz) tomato paste

☐

1 tablespoon dried basil leaves

☐

1 teaspoon dried oregano leaves

☐

1 tablespoon sugar

☐

1/2 teaspoon salt

☐

1/2 teaspoon pepper

⁇
1/2 teaspoon crushed red pepper flakes

Directions:

1.
Spray 5-quart slow cooker with cooking spray. In 12-inch skillet, cook sausage, onions, mushrooms and garlic over medium heat about 10 minutes, stirring occasionally, until sausage is no longer pink; drain.

2.
Spoon sausage mixture into cooker. Stir in remaining ingredients. Cover; cook on Low heat setting 8 to 9 hours.

Spicy Hamburger Goulash

Ingredients

- 1 pound ground beef

- 4 cans (14.5 ounces) diced tomatoes

- 1 can (4 ounces) diced green chilies

- 1 ½ cups cooked pinto beans

- 1 ½ cups cooked navy beans

- ½ cup chopped onion

- ½ cup chopped green pepper

- 2 tablespoons chili powder 1 teaspoon cumin

- 1 tablespoon Worcestershire sauce

- 2 teaspoons beef bouillon granules

- 1 teaspoon dried basil

⬚

¼ teaspoon white pepper

⬚

2 cups broken noodles

Directions:

1.

Brown your hamburger in a skillet. Transfer to a greased crock.

2.

Stir in tomatoes, chilies, beans, onion, green pepper, chili powder, cumin, Worcestershire, beef bouillon, basil, and white pepper.

3.

Cover and cook on low for five hours.

4.

Stir in broken up noodles.

5.

Return lid and cook an additional 30 minutes or until noodles are tender.

Taco Meat

Ingredients

- ½ pound ground hamburger, browned

- 2 cups frozen corn

- ½ cup chopped onion

- 1 can (14.5 ounces) diced tomatoes with green chilies

- 1 can (8 ounces) tomato sauce

- 1 teaspoon cumin

- 1 teaspoon chili powder

- 1 cup black beans, cooked

- Taco salad fixings: lettuce, chips, shredded cheese, sour cream

Directions

1.

Combine the meat, corn, onion, tomatoes, tomato sauce, and seasonings in your greased crock pot. Stir well.

2.

Cover and cook on low for 3 hours.

3.

Add black beans and stir.

4.

Turn off crock pot and let mixture sit to warm beans.

5.

Serve meat on top of a taco salad.

Sweet 'n Sour Pork

Ingredients

-
4 Whole yellow onions, halved and sliced

-
4-6 cloves of garlic, crushed and divided

-
1 bay leaf

-
1 Teaspoon black pepper

-
3 Pound boneless pork shoulder or butt, cut into 1 inch cubes

-
1/2 Cup apple cider vinegar

-
1/2 Cup lite soy sauce

-
1 Tablespoon sugar or sugar substitute

Directions

1.

Spread half of the onions in bottom of slow cooker. Add 2 garlic cloves, the bay leaf and pepper.

2.

Arrange pork in a single layer on top of onions. Top with remaining onions and garlic.

3.

Drizzle vinegar and soy cause over all and sprinkle with sugar.

4.

Cover and cook on HIGH for 4 hours or LOW for 8 hours.

Cranberry Apple Stuffed Pork Loin

Ingredients

⬚

3-4 pound pork loin

⬚

Apple jelly

⬚

1/4 teaspoon dried rosemary

⬚

Dried cranberries

⬚

1/2 cup apple cider or juice

⬚

2 tablespoons Worcestershire sauce

⬚

2 tablespoons apple jelly

Directions:

1.

Cut your pork loin in half lengthwise.

2.

Cover the inside with apple jelly. Sprinkle the top with rosemary.

3.

Layer dried cranberries on one side of the pork loin. Fold over and tie together.

4.

Place the loin into the crockpot with ½ a cup of apple cider or juice and a tablespoon of Worchester sauce.

5.

Combine two tablespoons of jelly and mix with one tablespoon of Worchester sauce. Cover the pork loin with your mixture.

6.

For less than 3 lbs, I cook for 1.5 hours at high per lb of meat. For a 3-4 lb pork loin, I cook on low for 6 hours or high for 5 hours. Temperature should read 145 degrees.

Easy Crock Pot Ribs

Ingredients

- 5 pounds ribs, any style

- 2 teaspoons garlic powder

- 2 teaspoons onion powder

- 2 teaspoons chili powder

- 1 teaspoon salt

- 6 tablespoons sucanat (or brown sugar)

- 5 tablespoons ketchup

- ¼ cup water

- ½ teaspoon Worcestershire sauce

- ½ teaspoon dry mustard

- ½ teaspoon paprika

- 1 teaspoon salt

- ¼ teaspoon pepper

- 4 tablespoons cornstarch

- 4 tablespoons water

Directions:

1.
Combine garlic powder, onion powder, chili powder, and 1 teaspoon salt. Rub into meat.

2.
Lay ribs in the bottom of a 5-6 quart greased crock pot. Layer if necessary.

3.
Combine sucanat, ketchup, water, Worcestershire, mustard, paprika, salt, and pepper. Whisk to combine.

4.
Pour over meat.

5.
Cover and cook on low for 8 hours – until meat has a temperature of 170 degrees.

6.
Remove meat from crock and keep warm.

7.
Skim grease from sauce if desired (I don't).

8.

Combine cornstarch and water. Stir into juices.

9.

Cover and cook on HIGH for 30 minutes or until thickened. Serve sauce over meat.

Pasta with Pork Ragu

Ingredients

-
1 carrot, large, chopped

-
1 onion, medium, chopped

-
1 garlic clove, chopped

-
2 T. tomato paste

-
2 tsp. thyme, dried

-
1 tsp. oregano, dried

-
Kosher salt and black pepper

-
14.5 oz. tomatoes, diced, canned

-
1 1/2 lb. pork, boneless, shoulder or butt, trimmed and cut in half

-
3/4 lb. fettuccini

-
Grated Parmesan, for serving

Directions:

1.

In a 4-6 quart slow cooker, combine the carrot, onion, garlic, tomato paste, thyme, oregano, 3/4 tsp. salt, and 1/4 tsp. pepper.

2.

Add the tomatoes (and the juices); add the pork and turn to coat.

3.

Cover. Cook on Low for 7-8 hours or on High for 5-6 hours, or until the pork is very tender.

4.

Twenty minutes before serving, cook the fettuccine according to the directions on the package, drain and return to the pot.

5.

Meanwhile, using 2 forks, shred the pork and mix it into the cooking liquid.

6.

Toss the pasta with the Ragu and sprinkle with Parmesan.

Parmesan Honey Pork Roast

Ingredients

- 2 - 3 lbs. pork roast, boneless

- 2/3 c. Parmesan cheese, grated

- 1/2 c. honey

- 3 T. soy sauce

- 2 T. basil, dried

- 2 T. garlic, minced

- 2 T. olive oil

- 1/2 tsp. salt

- Gravy:

- 2 T. cornstarch

- 1/4 c. water, cold

Directions:

1.

Spray slow cooker with non-stick cooking spray.

2.

Place roast in slow cooker.

3.

In a bowl, combine cheese, honey, soy sauce, basil, garlic, oil and salt; pour over pork.

4.

Cover. Cook on Low for 6-7 hours or until a meat thermometer reads 160°.

5.

Remove pork to a serving platter; keep warm.

6.

Skim fat from cooking juices; transfer to a small saucepan. Bring liquid to a boil.

7.

Combine cornstarch and water until smooth.

8.

Gradually stir into pan. Bring to a boil; cook and stir for 2 minutes or until thickened.

Mexican Pork Roast

Ingredients

- 1 2-lb. pork roast

- 1 small onion, peeled, ends removed, sliced

- 2 cloves garlic, minced or grated

- 1 c. water

- 1 tbsp. cumin

- 1 tbsp. chili powder

- ¼ tsp. black pepper

- 1 tsp. sea salt

- 1 cup dry pinto or black beans, soaked overnight

Directions

1.

Add everything to the crockpot and cook 3 – 4 hours on high, or 6 – 8 hours on low.

2.

Before serving, use two forks to pull the meat apart.

3.

You can use a slotted spoon to remove the beans from the crockpot first (if, for example, you have some family members who don't care for them), or you can mix it all together.

4.

 Serve over lettuce, or put in tortillas.

5.

Makes 6 – 8 servings.

Pork Roast with Apples & Sweet Potatoes

Ingredients

- lb pork roast

- 2 fuji apples, cored and chopped

- medium sweet potato, chopped in large pieces

- medium onion, chopped in large pieces

- tbsp minced garlic

- cup apple juice (or white grape juice or water)

- tsp sea salt

- ½ tsp black pepper

- ½ tsp ground cinnamon

- ½ tsp dried basil

-

½ tsp dried rosemary

-

½ tsp dried marjoram

-

¼ - ½ tsp crushed red pepper flakes (to taste)

Directions:

1.
Spray the bottom and sides of a 4.5 quart slow cooker.

2.
Place half of the apple, sweet potato, and onion chunks in the bottom of the slow cooker. Place the roast on top, followed by the juice.

3.
Sprinkle the herbs and spices over the roast, followed by the remaining chunks of apple, sweet potato and onion. Cover and cook on low for 6-8 hours or high for 3.5 – 4.5 hours.

4.
Once finished, remove and slice the pork roast. Scoop the apple, sweet potato, and onion chunks into a bowl and mash with a potato masher.

5.
Serves 4

Smothered Chops with Onions and Bacon

Ingredients:

- 4 ounces bacon (about 4 slices), chopped

- 3 onions, halved and sliced ½ inch thick

- 4 teaspoons brown sugar

- 3 garlic cloves, minced

- tablespoon minced fresh thyme or 1 teaspoon dried

- ⅓ cup all-purpose flour

- cup low-sodium chicken broth

- ¼ cup soy sauce

- bay leaves

- 6 7-ounce bone-in blade-cut pork chops, about ¾ inch thick, sides slit to prevent curling

-

Salt and pepper

-

tablespoon cider vinegar

-

tablespoon minced fresh parsley

Directions:

1.

Cook bacon in 12-inch skillet over medium heat until crisp, 5 to 7 minutes; transfer to slow cooker. Pour off all but 2 tablespoons bacon fat left in skillet.

2.

Add onions, 1 teaspoon sugar, garlic, and thyme to fat in skillet and cook over medium-high heat until onions are softened and well browned, about 10 minutes. Stir in flour and cook for 1 minute. Slowly whisk in broth, scraping up any browned bits and smoothing out and lumps; transfer to slow cooker.

3.

Stir remaining tablespoon sugar, soy sauce, and bay leaves into slow cooker. Season pork chops with salt and pepper and nestle into slow cooker. Cover and cook until pork is tender, 6 to 8 hours on low or 3 to 5 hours on high.

4.

Transfer pork chops to serving platter, tent loosely with aluminum foil, and let rest for 10 minutes.

5.

Let braising liquid settle for 5 minutes, then remove fat from surface using large spoon.

6.

Discard bay leaves. Stir in vinegar and parsley and season with salt and pepper to taste. Spoon 1 cup sauce over chops and serve with remaining sauce.

Sweet Balsamic Glazed Pork Loin

YIELD: SERVES 6-8

Ingredients

Pork:

- 2 pound boneless pork loin roast, trimmed of large fat pockets

- 1 teaspoon ground sage

- 1/2 teaspoon salt

- 1/2 teaspoon pepper

- 1 clove garlic, finely minced or crushed

- 1/2 cup water

Glaze:

- 1/2 cup brown sugar, light or dark

- 1 tablespoon cornstarch

- 1/4 cup balsamic vinegar

-

1/2 cup water

-

2 tablespoons soy sauce

Directions:

1.
In a small bowl, combine the sage, salt, pepper and garlic.

2.
Rub the spices all over the roast.

3.
Place the pork roast in the slow cooker and pour in the 1/2 cup water. Cover and cook on low for 6-8 hours.

4.
Near the end of the cooking time for the roast, combine the ingredients for the glaze in a small saucepan and bring the mixture to a boil, then reduce and let the mixture simmer, stirring occasionally, until it thickens.

5.
Remove the pork from the slow cooker, shred and place on a platter or plate. Drizzle the glaze over the pork and serve.

Salt Crusted Pork Roast

Ingredients

-

2-3 pound Pork Sirloin Roast

Seasoning Blend

-

1 Tablespoon salt

-

1 Tablespoon black pepper

-

1 teaspoon garlic powder

-

1 teaspoon paprika

-

1 teaspoon dry sweet basil

-

1 teaspoon ground sage

Instructions

1.

Mix the seasoning blend together in a small bowl

2.

Pat dry the roast and rub seasoning blend into meat, coating well

3.

Brown the roast on the stove top over medium heat, 2-3 minutes on all sides until you get a nice carmelization

4.

Cook in a slow cooker for 8 hours on the keep warm setting until internal temperature is 145 F

5.

Remove from cooker and allow to rest for 5-10 minutes before slicing

Ham, Green Beans, & Potatoes

Ingredients

SERVINGS 6-8

*

1smoked pork hock

*

1(15 ounce) jarwhole white pearl onions

*

1(16 ounce) packagecooked diced ham (or leftover sliced ham)

*

1(16 ounce) bag frozen French-cut green beans (or regular cut, or canned)

*

4baking potatoes, diced (or red potatoes, halved)

Directions:

1.

Combine all ingredients in crock pot. (There's no need to defrost any ingredients that have been frozen.).

2.

Cook on low for 6 hours.

BACON & CHEESE QUICHE

Ingredients

- 1 tablespoon butter

- 10 eggs, beaten

- 1 cup light cream or half & half

- 8 ounces shredded cheddar cheese

- ½ teaspoon black pepper

- 10 pieces cooked bacon, chopped

- ½ cup chopped spinach

Directions:

1.

Grease the slow cooker crock with the butter (leave excess in the crock); set aside.

2.

In a large mixing bowl, combine the eggs, cream, cheese, spinach and pepper, then add to the slow cooker.

3.

Sprinkle the cooked bacon over the top of the mixture.

4.

Cover and cook on LOW for 4 hours.

5.

Keep an eye on it. Do not overcook or the quiche will be dry.

Bacon-Wrapped Pork Loin Roast

Ingredients

-
1 1/2 to 2 lb pork loin roast

-
6 to 8 slice bacon, uncooked

-
salt and pepper to taste

Directions:

1.
Wash pork roast and pat dry.

2.
Add salt and pepper to taste.

3.
Wrap pork roast in uncooked bacon slices, securing underneath the roast.

4.
Cook in crockpot on low heat for about 5 to 6 hours or until bacon is cooked and roast is tender.

5.
Transfer to serving platter.

6.
Pour broth into a sauce pan and bring to a boil.

7.

Thicken using about 2 teaspoons of cornstarch mixed with enough milk to make a pourable paste. Add cornstarch mixture to broth a little at a time, whisking constantly .

SWEET & SPICY PORK PICADILLO

Ingredients

- 1 TBSP olive oil

- 1 Diced Yellow Onion

- 2 cloves minced garlic

- 1 lb boneless pork country style ribs cut into 1 inch cubes

- 1 can (14 oz) diced tomatoes undrained

- 3 tbsp cider vinegar

- 2 chipotle peppers in adobe sauce chopped (optional)

- ½ cup raisins chopped

- ½ tsp cumin

- ½ tsp ground cinnamon

- salt and pepper to taste

Directions:

1.

Heat oil in skilled over medium low heat until hot. Cook and Stir onion and garlic until translucent about 4 minutes.

2.

Add pork to skillet an brown. Transfer to crockpot

3.

Combine Tomatoes with juice, vinegar, chipotles, raisins, cumin & cinnamon in medium bowl. Pour over pork.

4.

Cover and cook on low 5 hours or high 3 hours. or until pork is fork tender.

5.

Shred pork using 2 forks. Cook 30 minutes longer. Adjust seasonings before serving with rice.

Lamb Curry

Ingredients

▢
1 ½ pound lamb (leave in large pieces, so it will be easier to remove) chicken and beef are also a good substitute

▢
1 large onion, diced

▢
2 garlic cloves, minced

▢
3 tablespoons curry powder (ours has ground coriander, turmeric, cumin, fenugreek, yellow mustard, white pepper, ginger, cinnamon, chili powder, cloves, cardamom, fennel)

▢
1 teaspoon garam masala

▢
Salt and pepper

▢
½ cup sour cream, yogurt or buttermilk

Directions:

1.
Put the onions and garlic in the crock pot and stir in the curry powder and garam masala.

2.

Add the meat and sprinkle with a little more curry powder and some salt and pepper.

3.

Cook on high 1 hour and then low 5 hours.

4.

Carefully remove the meat and then puree the onions, garlic and meat juices with an immersion blender.

5.

Shred the meat (removing any bones!) and return it to the crockpot.

6.

Stir in the sour cream (or yogurt or buttermilk) and add more curry powder, salt or pepper, as needed.

7.

Serve over rice or couscous.

Seafood Paella

Ingredients:

- 3/4 c. chopped sweet peppers

- 1/2 c. chopped onion

- 2 cloves garlic, minced

- 2 1/2 cups chicken broth

- 1 c. uncooked brown rice

- 1/2 tsp. dried thyme

- 1/4 tsp. crushed red pepper

- 1/4 tsp. ground tumeric

- 12 oz. fresh or frozen shrimp, thawed, peeled and halved

- 6 oz. canned or pouched wild-caught pink salmon, flaked

- 1 c. frozen peas

Method:

1.

Grease crock pot and add all veggies except peas. In a medium sauce pan, combine chicken broth, rice and spices.

2.

Heat until boiling, then pour over veggies in the crock pot. Cover and cook on low for 4 hours.

3.

After about 3 hours, add the shrimp, salmon and peas. Once done, let stand for about 10 minutes before serving.

4.

Serves 6.

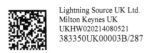